Somatic Gratitude

MANTRAS & GRATITUDE MEDITATIONS TO FOSTER BODY POSITIVITY & SELF-LOVE

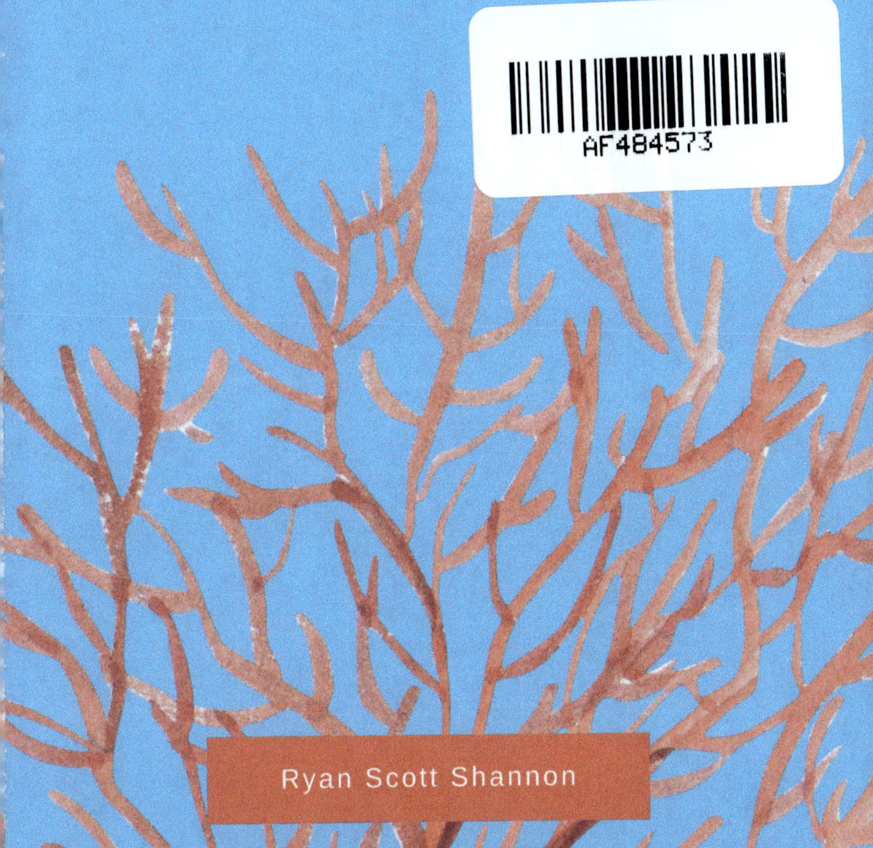

Ryan Scott Shannon

Disclaimer: This book is not intended for the purpose of providing medical advice. All information, content, and material of this book is for informational purposes only and are not intended to serve as a substitute for the consultation, diagnosis, and/or medical treatment of a qualified physician or healthcare provider.

Table of Contents

Get Out Of Fight-or-Flight Mode and Into a State of Gratitude

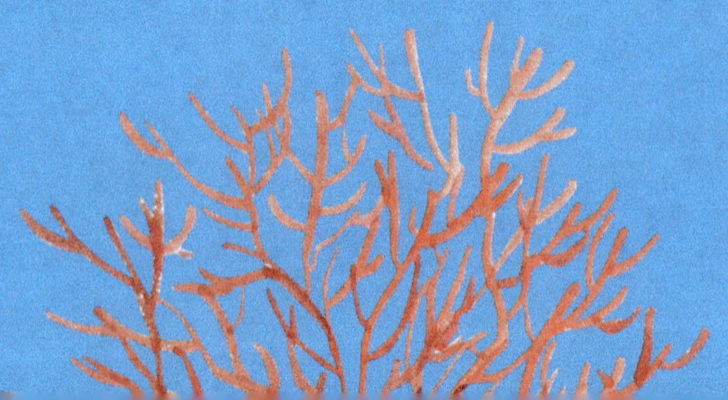

Learning to Love Ourselves & Our Bodies

Do you feel uncomfortable living in your body?
Do you find yourself focusing on wanting to change parts of your physical self?
Do you avoid looking in the mirror, or on the flipside, obsessive gaze upon your reflection?

We enter the world, occupying a body, through no choice of our own. And yet, somehow, for many of us, we haven't quite accepted this fleshy thing we live in and the way we feel about it. While feelings and attitudes towards our bodies may be ever-changing, it's easy to gravitate toward the negative spectrum of emotions. We may despair at the appearance of fine lines. We may feel hopeless as the number on the scale never seems to decrease. We may feel betrayed when our face flushes upon looking at our crush. We may even feel damaged beyond repair upon receiving a chronic illness diagnosis.

While it's important to feel a full spectrum of emotions and avoid suppressing our authentic feelings, it's equally important to "unstuck" ourselves. That is, we can step out of the negative self-images we've created and choose to erase our attachment to these (often false and distorted) images. We can change our thoughts and attitudes towards the parts of ourselves that are seemingly unlovable, and we can change our behavior, too. The goal of this guide is to empower you (there's so much within your control!) and help you radiate with love towards yourself (and, consequently, others).

How do we erase false images of ourselves? For example, you may feel despair initially when seeing crow's feet form at the corner of your eyes. But guess what? Getting older is a privilege! So many of us die before we even have an opportunity to form. Not only, but crow's feet are also the result of smiling and laughter—a few lines at the corner of the eyes are a small price to pay for laughter and smiles. These reframings, borrowed from Cognitive Behavior Therapy (CBT) are sprinkled throughout this guide and can help you find a new appreciation for the body you live in.

Beyond just changing our thoughts, I also wanted to emphasize the power of changing our behavior. If there's something about ourselves that's impacting our self-esteem, or is leading to the degradation of our health, then it's important to not only reframe thoughts but to take action. Continuing with the crow's feet example, you may decide that you'd like to prevent, and possibly reverse, them from becoming deeper by means of retinol, mineral-based SPF, and a good moisturizer. You may even cut the sugar and processed seed oils— two ingredients known to expedite the breakdown of collagen. You'll notice a common theme throughout this guide is the striving for equilibrium between accepting and loving the parts of ourselves we can't change (via reframing) and taking action on the parts of ourselves we can change (via behavioral changes).

Ultimately, the power lies in your hands. These mantras will help you to feel love, gratitude, and even awe towards the unchangeable parts of your physical self, and determined, empowered, and focused on taking the necessary actions to evoke positive change. While reflecting on these mantras, and doing the mindfulness-inspired activities, it should become easier for you to decide what's unchangeable and what you have the power to change.

To reiterate, this mantra-centered guide is an opportunity for you to reframe your perception of your body. Rather than engaging with inflammatory emotions directed at yourself, these mantras invite you to pivot. Now, you can turn away from resentment, and focus on gratitude. You can banish apathy, and cultivate self-compassion. You can reject self-destruction, and instead surrender yourself to the best version of yourself.

It's time to experience somatic gratitude. Settle into a quiet, comfortable setting to explore yourself and shift your emotional state through these mantras.

Introduction to Mantras

Are you feeling unmotivated when it comes to your health goals?
Do you feel like your beliefs hold you back from being a better you?
Are you tired of not making meaningful changes that stick?

If so, mantras can help you! There's convincing research that mediation techniques, including the use of mantras, can help reduce stress and possibly help you make more rationa,l objective decisions. If you'd like to help reprogram your inner beliefs so that they better suit your healing goals, then this is the book for you.

This book is split up into four main sections: 1. Creating change right here, right now 2. Future self-visualizations 3. Radical gratitude and awe, and 4. Entrusting the mysteries and science of the body. These four sections combine to help overhaul your current beliefs surrounding your body and hopefully replace them with the belief that you are strong, capable of change and accepting of your body no matter its condition.

Within each section, you'll receive several mantras as well as a breakdown to help you better digest them. These mantras can be spoken aloud to yourself in a quiet room or can be read and reread in your head.

Not only, you'll also be given mindfulness-infused exercises after receiving each mantra to help the mantra "stick". These exercises are inspired by "Anapana" and "Vipassana" meditation techniques that help you to realize everything is transient, including the negative feelings you may harbor towards yourself and your body.

I hope this book of mantras is insightful, inspiring, and leads to positive changes in your life.

Mantras... Quackery? Or an Effective Strategy to Train the Brain?

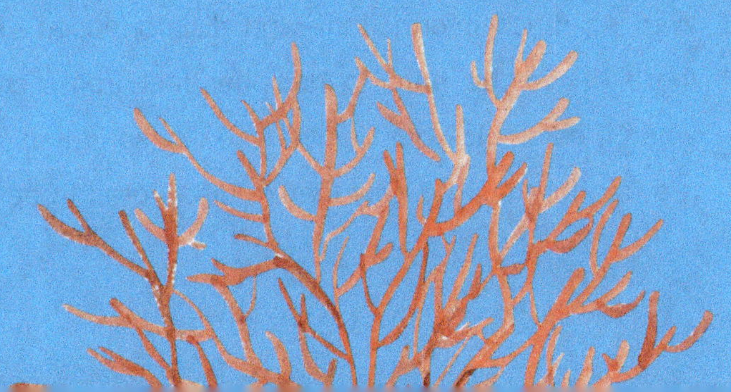

Mantras…Quackery? Or an Effective Strategy to Train the Brain?

Wait, how can mantras help you heal? You may be asking yourself this question. While it may seem like quackery, there is some convincing evidence that supports the effectiveness of mantras. Reciting mantras can help reduce symptoms of post-traumatic stress disorder, manage stress, and build resilience (Oman et al. 2022). And meditation, in general, has a range of benefits that you may be aware of, including: decreased blood pressure, even in those with hypertension; increased energy levels; better immune system function (Hyland et al., 2015); and even improved work satisfaction (Hülsheger & Alberts, 2020).

With so much information—and disinformation—out there, it can be hard to decipher fact from fiction when it comes to your health. One day saturated fats are bad for you, the next they're discovered to be an important fatty acid found in human breast milk and a necessary precursor to sex hormones like testosterone, estrogen, and progesterone. One day cholesterol clogs the arteries, the next it's necessary for maintaining cell membranes, acts as a precursor to vitamin D production, and can help repair inflammation-induced damage.

With so much flip-flopping, how can you be sure mantras will be beneficial to you? First, mantras have been safely and effectively used for thousands of years in both Eastern and Western cultures. Next, the scientific literature on mantras, prayer and meditation is robust (more on this in the upcoming section).

I don't mean to add to the confusion by mentioning these health contradictions that are spouted off at us. Rather, I hope to show you that the ultimate power lies in you. You decide what goes into your body. You decide what you value. You decide what's credible. You're the ultimate authority over your life. Whether that means resorting to the analytical mind and combing through PubMed to find studies that support a hypothesis you've built up in your mind, or simply relying on deep-seated intuition, the solutions lie within you.

Let these mantras be a way to help you rediscover your innate healing capabilities and put your mind at ease. I hope these serve as tools to help you return to a state of ease rather than disease.

Sorting Through the Chaos

You may be wondering how reciting some words a few times a day will make a difference in your journey towards better health and becoming a better you. While it may seem very *woo-woo*, mantras can help you access your highest self. The self that helps you navigate the ever-changing health fads and misinformation.

Regular repetition will create new connections in the brain, allowing you to kick your old habits that have been encoded into the subconscious mind. In fact, this idea is supported by a study on mantras and PTSD among war veterans; it was found that a higher frequency of mantra practice was associated with better clinical outcomes, including less severe PTSD symptoms and decreased anger ([Malaktaris et al, 2022](#)). In essence, by utilizing mantras, you'll be upgrading your subconscious mind with new, higher values.

It's thought that in our infancy (ages zero to six) we're nothing but sponges. This is when our programming is installed. Everything from the language we speak, to the way we form romantic relationships (i.e. Attachment Style Theory), to personality is thought to be encoded during this critical life stage. You've probably received some programming throughout your life (especially from childhood) that has influenced your values—and not for the better.

Remember those fast food commercials that would play during your favorite cartoons? Your favorite athletes' faces on sugary cereals? The magazines that tricked you into believing there are shortcuts and miracle pills to help keep you thin? These are just a few examples of the way predatory marketing practices and lax government regulation may have tarnished your subconscious mind and values.

Sadly, many involved in pharmaceuticals (including immoral doctors) have a vested interest in dissuading the masses. Whistleblower Carlat, M.D. reveals in his book, "Unhinged: The Trouble with Psychiatry" that many other psychiatrists push ineffective drugs rather than practice psychotherapy. More sick people on drugs means more money. As of now, the total nominal spending on pharmaceuticals in 2019 was 511.4 billion dollars (Statista, 2019).

Unlike many doctors, I'm not selling you anything. Rather, my goal in writing these mantras and disseminating this information to you is to help you and others make positive changes on a micro level so that we all benefit at a macro level.

In other words, when you make your health and bettering your life a priority, you're playing a key role in making the world a better place. Unlike those pesky commercials for medications that are constantly aired on TV, I make virtually no money from the information I provide (just a few dollars). There's no financial incentive for me to write this book; I'm doing it to help you help yourself.

Now, before we start reciting mantras, I want to go over why mantras can help you. There's no way mantras can have powerful physiological effects on the body, right?

Turns out, they can!

Reciting a few words throughout the day with intention will almost magically help you upgrade the current version of yourself. *Abrakadabra!* This popular, magical phrase stems from Aramaic, meaning "I will create as I speak." Your words, mantras, and prayers are powerful spells that direct your actions (that's why you should always be careful of how you speak of yourself and others).

Now, let's cover the science of mantras.

The Science Behind Mantras, Prayers & Meditations

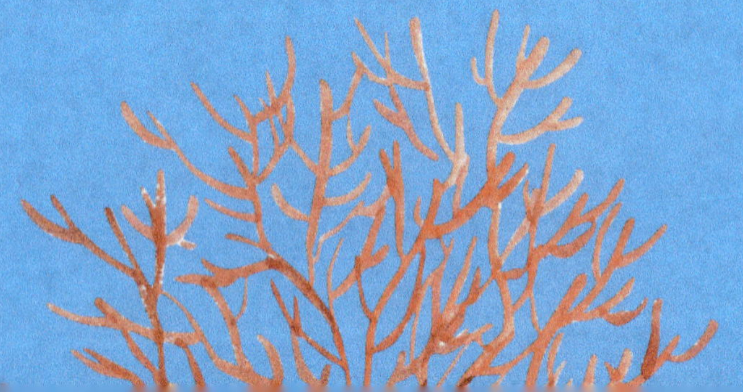

The Science Behind Mantras, Prayers, and Affirmations

To believe something, it's got to make sense. While it may seem crazy to think that meditation and mantras can lead to a better body and health, you'll understand through the following summaries of studies how reduced stress, lowered inflammation, and increased cognition can lead to a better you. The studies prove mantras, meditation and prayers are highly effective in achieving physical changes—it really may be mind over matter after all!

Mantras are similar to prayers in that they're both typically short statements that help you to align with higher values that are usually said throughout the day. I decided to use 'mantra' in the title rather than 'prayer' since 'mantra' doesn't have a religious connotation, however, we can think of them as almost the same. Instead of the "Hail Mary" for Catholics, the "Shema" for Jews, and the "Shahada" for Muslims, mantras can be thought of as universal prayers for those of any—or no—religious affiliation.

- **Significant brain changes were found in 78 studies**. In a meta-analysis, neuroimaging studies involving the brain activity of subjects while meditating (which included mantra meditation) were compared to control groups. This meta-analysis concluded that the "insula, frontopolar cortex and dorsal anterior cingulate" were all activated during meditation (Fox et al, 2016).

- **Curbs cortisol which is associated with chronic inflammation, depression and disease**. Cortisol has entered common parlance in recent years for good reason. While cortisol is an important hormone necessary for sustaining life and repairing trauma to the body, too much of a good thing can be bad. One study notes that "*heightened inflammatory cytokine levels driven by stress may contribute to depression symptoms by contributing to cell death in brain regions involved in the regulation of mood and emotion*" (Pascoe et al, 2021). Fortunately, meditation has been shown to lower cortisol ([Hopper et al., 2019](#))

- **Meditation may boost the immune system.** One study involving 30 women found that those who meditated had levels of Immunoglobulin A (IgA, an important protein created by the immune system to find and neutralize pathogens) that were significantly different from those who didn't meditate: "The mean s-IgA titer in the experimental group at 'post-meditation' and '1-hour later' time-points were found to be statistically different from those of the control group" ([Torkamani et al, 2018](#)). In other words, mantra meditation may lead to better immunological outcomes.

- **Meditation can change the way you perceive stressors.** This meta-study found important changes in self-compassion, stress response, and other parameters: "Meditation practices are shown to influence many psychological processes that can influence an individual's psychological response and relationship with stressors, including self-compassion, rumination, exposure, metacognition and attention" (Pascoe et al, 2021). Through meditation and mantras, you will shape the way you perceive any health issues you may have. A change in perception and less stress may result in better decision-making and steps in the right direction.

In summary, by meditating on these mantras, you'll hopefully greatly reduce your stress levels, decrease chronic inflammation loads, lessen anger, and even alleviate symptoms of trauma. The many exercises will help you feel grounded, placing you in a state that's more receptive to each mantra.

How to Get the Most Out of This Book

This isn't a work of fiction. It's not a self-help book (although you may find help from reading this book). This is a tool to help you access your inner core and speak to it so that you can make changes in your life that make you a stronger, healthier you. You can jump around from section to section, you can come back to certain mantras, and you can even skip over mantras that don't speak to you.

The point is to leverage this book so that it works for you—maybe you will read the book through in its entirety, or maybe you just prioritize the sections that are most relevant to you. In general, to reap the benefits of the mantras, it's important that you follow some (or all) of the following six steps.

1. **Repeat, repeat, repeat.** When learning anything, it's important to employ a strategy that leverages "spaced repetitions." In other words, it's important to expose yourself to

these mantras more than just once or twice. To truly learn something, you've got to repeat reviews over a period of time. For example, you might read a mantra and re-read it the following day, then the next week, then the following week thereafter.

2. **Keep an open mind.** It's important to question your beliefs. Many have built their identities around beliefs that may not be true, or that may be more nuanced than previously realized. For example, you may believe "I'll always be unathletic." I'm asking you to keep an open mind. To be willing to push yourself. To expand or contract your definition of "athleticism", for example. Be open to change.

3. **Do the exercises.** Reading the mantras, and repeating them, can take you far, but the exercises can really help you to make meaningful changes. Most of the exercises are based on powerful meditation techniques I've acquired over the years and can help you find the stillness required to make changes.

4. **If you fall off course, remember you can come back to this book** (if you've only got the eBook, get the physical copy too. Keep it somewhere visible). Always remember that mistakes and poor decisions can arise. Forgive yourself quickly. You're human. Just remember you can pick this book back up again and start fresh. It may help to keep this book in a physical place to remind you of your commitment to change.

5. **Write it out on a piece of paper.** Writing things down can improve your retention. If there's a mantra that you just want to make stick, getting it down on your own piece of paper can be a great way to do so. Go ahead and grab your favorite pen, or colored pencils, and write down as plainly or creatively the mantras you'd like to adopt.

I hope this book inspires you to take actions that lead to a better you, all while lowering your stress levels and improving your sense of agency. You're capable of change, and I hope you adopt this belief throughout this process. Now, it's time to dig into some mantras!

Radical Appreciation and Awe

Practicing Gratitude

Have you ever written a thank you letter to your body? That may sound odd but just think of all the amazing things your body does for you. It transports you (have you ever thought about how depressing and unfulfilling it'd be to not be able to transport yourself with your body? To never move?). It tells you when it's hungry. Sometimes hunger can be annoying, but think about it for a moment. If you didn't have these hunger signals, you'd starve to death. Thank your grumbling stomach the next time you go without food!

Your body even rewards you with feelings of pleasure which is important for everything from raising children to creating social bonds. Our bodies conspire to make us feel good when we exercise (hello, endorphins!) and when we achieve something (accomplishment can even stimulate the production of testosterone). Further, our bodies even grow strong when we stress them with stimulus— be it physical or mental. Our bodies are constructed in a way that protects our organs. Our bodies are equipped with autonomic processes that help us in times of stress.

Have you ever thought of muscle growth as a miracle? When you stress your muscles by lifting heavy objects (i.e. weights), you're breaking down muscle fibers. Once you rest and provide the body with adequate nourishment, muscles should develop. But what happens if your routine gets out of whack and you take your training too far? The body goes into "protective mode" if you exercise too much. Let's say you're going to the gym lifting heavy for 2 hours a day most days of the week but are only sleeping 5 hours. Your body will respond by increasing fat storage and increasing cortisol production (which suppresses appetite and lowers inflammation, at least in the short-term) and you'll likely feel fatigued and sore.

This condition, known as overtraining, is yet another example of your body trying to help you reach that perfect equilibrium. Too much of a good thing (like exercise) can lead to bad effects. Fortunately, our body is constantly sending us signals to guide us back on the right path. We just have to listen.

These signals are sent to us unconsciously, meaning we have no awareness or control over this process. It comes entirely from the "software" of our very intelligent bodies. And for that, we should be tremendously grateful!

I Am Grateful
for This Body
That I Live In

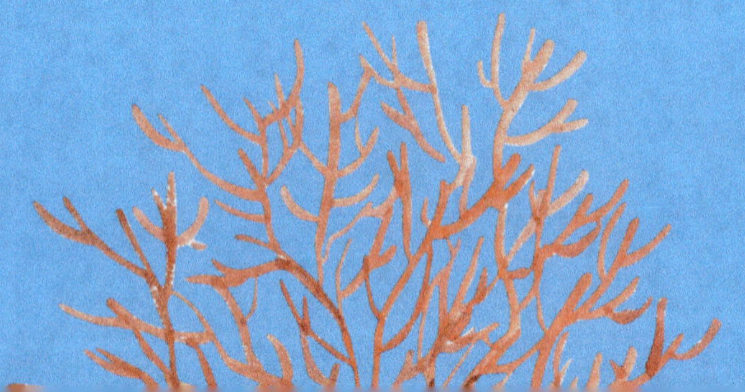

I Am Grateful for this Body that I Live In

What if you were to express deep gratitude for your body, through which you're able to experience sensations and interact with the world? As mentioned, your body does lots of cool things for you. It's your vehicle, allowing you to drive through life. It's your avatar. It's your vessel for the soul. It's your home.

Instead of complaining about what your body doesn't do or how it doesn't look, try focusing your attention on what it does and how it actually looks. Even if it's something small; run with it. You could be grateful for waking up today. Grateful for your beating heart. Grateful for the fact that your body has innate protective mechanisms like shivering, which helps keep the body warm, or fever, which increases the body's internal temperature to help kill off bacteria and even viruses.

When we learn to be grateful for the tremendous bodies we live in, our journey toward healthy living becomes easier. Try to find a different reason to be grateful for your body each time you read this mantra. Try to think with an abundance mindset: 'It's hard to find just one reason to be grateful!' There is so much to be grateful for!

Embody this Mantra:

1. Close your eyes in a quiet room.
2. Breathe in fully through your eyes.
3. Pause briefly and feel gratitude for the body you live in.
4. Exhale and repeat the process a few times.
5. After completing the exercise, affirm to yourself "I am grateful for my body, my home"

My Body Communicates Signals to Me and I'm Grateful For This Dialogue

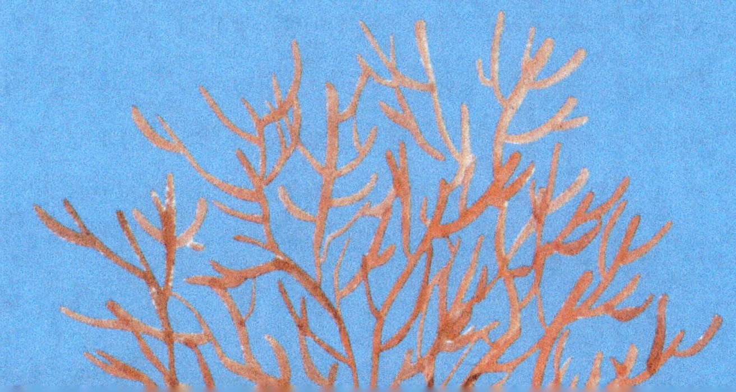

My Body Communicates Signals to Me and I'm Grateful For This Dialogue

Sure, hunger can be uncomfortable (though, there's plenty of research that demonstrates intermittent fasting i.e. eating for a restricted time period each day, has immense anti-cancer, longevity, and inflammation-quelching benefits) but without this signal, we would starve to death. Think of it as a necessary evil. The sensation of hunger can be uncomfortable, but it's our innate drive to seek out food. Similar primal urges push us to drink water, find a mate, sleep and so on.

There are many examples of our body communicating its needs to us. Anxiety is another example. Did you know anxiety can actually be a good thing? And that without anxiety, you probably wouldn't achieve much? Virtually everyone experiences anxiety to some degree. It can be felt before approaching deadlines, before delivering a speech, and before going on a date with someone you're attracted to. While anxiety can feel debilitating in some cases, it's purported that anxiety is necessary to accomplish goals and may even indicate higher emotional intelligence.

There are many somatic signals that seem to be working against us, but really, the body is pushing us toward our higher selves. With this mantra, let gratitude flow over you as you reflect on the dialogue you have with your body.

Embody this Mantra:

1. Sit comfortably on a chair or the floor.
2. Begin to focus your attention on the sensation of breathing. You may notice the rise and fall of your belly, the sensation of the breath passing through your nose, the expansion of your rib cage.
3. As you begin feeling your breath, take into account other sensations in your body. Allow your attention to hone in on a sensation that arises, and once it changes or subsides, draw your attention to a new sensation.

4. After spending some time feeling sensations, tell yourself "I am grateful for the signals I receive from my body)

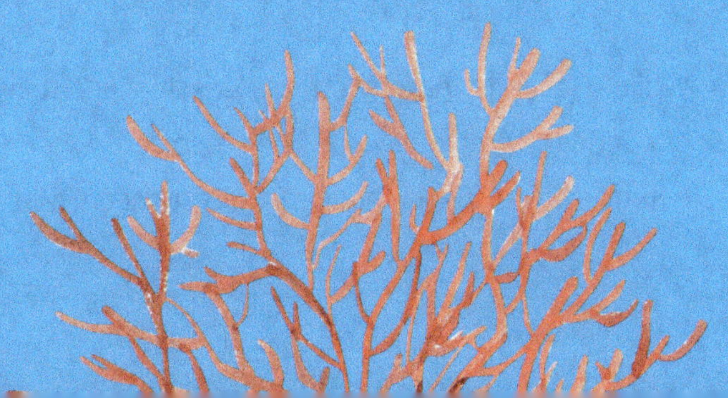

I Respect My
Body and Allow
It to Guide Me
to Equilibrium

I Respect My Body and Allow It to Guide Me to Equilibrium

Sometimes our primal urges can push us off track, which is why we need to evaluate our signals with the intellect. Take cravings as an example. There may be times when we want anything out of a can, a package or from our favorite fast food restaurant (that we know isn't good for us). Instead of giving into cravings and animalistic urges, it's important to stop and think first.

Rather than being hungry, you may learn that you were actually instead thirsty (dehydration is known to be mistaken for hunger). If you decide to give into your craving anyway, indulging in a greasy fast food burger, you might listen closely to your body and realize that it gave you indigestion and a feeling of heat (inflammation).

While it sounds far-fetched and unscientific, many of our health problems can be resolved when we actually listen to our bodies in conjunction with the mind. This productive duo allows us to free ourselves from being enslaved by our taste buds. Learn to listen to these signals from your body, sorting out craving from necessity. Remember, your body's always working in your favor to seek equilibrium.

Embody this Mantra:

1. Close your eyes, or soften your gaze.
2. Take a deep breath all the way to your belly button.
3. Breathe out fully and recite "I choose to respect my body and allow it to guide me to optimal health." a few times (or as many as needed).

I Use My Free Will to Make Choices that Honor My Sacred Body

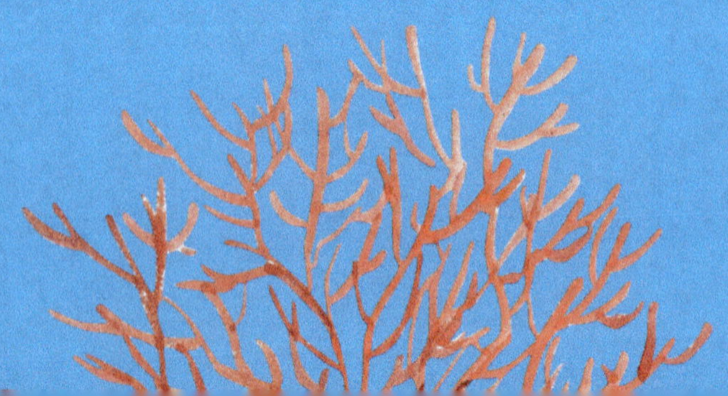

I Use My Free Will to Make Choices that Honor My Sacred Body

First, it can be argued we don't entirely have free will with what we put into our bodies. For example, living in a big city often means breathing in higher quantities of pollution— we don't have full control of breathing in PM 2.5 and other pollutants! Yes, we could hypothetically move, but for some, that's not viable. An additional example of a lack of free will are "food deserts" in the US, where some populations lack access to grocery stores. While food desert residents could bus to Costco and buy in bulk, or grow their own food, this isn't very practical.

Despite these challenges, there's still plenty that's within our hands. We can choose whether we opt for grass-fed beef or conventional. We can opt for uncured, free-range pork, or settle for bacon from inhumanely treated pigs.

We have the option to eat out, but we also have the option to eat in which is usually the healthier and more budget-friendly option. Astoundingly, per U.S. Bureau of Labor Statistics, the average American household spent an average of $3,450 per year on food away from home (i.e. restaurants and takeout) each year between 2017 and 2019 (2020) While there certainly are factors that impede our ability to act freely, it can be assumed we all have the ability to choose between eating in versus eating out. While eating out on occasion is fine, in excess it may hamper your ability to make meaningful changes to your physiology. Which wolf will you feed?

Embody this Mantra:

1. With this mantra, focus on feeding the positive part of yourself.
2. Entrust yourself to make the best decisions that feed your highest self.
3. Take a deep breath through your nose.
4. Hold your breath for three seconds.
5. As you exhale, imagine toxic black smoke exiting your nose representing choices that disrespect your body and well-being.

My Mind Is Constantly Guiding Me to Make Better Choices For My Health

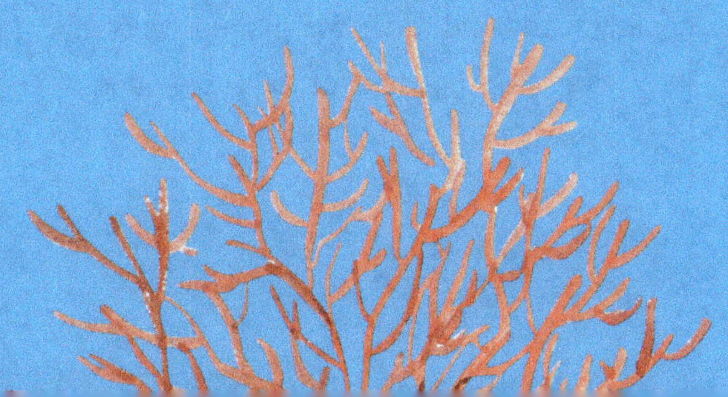

My Mind Is Constantly Guiding Me to Make Better Choices For My Health

Before reflecting on this mantra, cast an image of your ideal self in your mind. Take a moment to reflect on the physical and non-physical attributes of this person. What does it feel like to be your ideal self? As you probably know, it will require you to consciously change to become this ideal version of yourself. You've got to direct your energy toward the goal of reaching that ideal version that's alive in you. When that goal is placed at the forefront of your mind, you spend your time and resources towards achieving that goal, and it becomes a self-fulfilling prophecy.

When you focus on the positive outcome (that you can and will reach!) you are guiding your mind and body to seek out healing. You'll begin to be drawn to healthy foods and activities that upgrade your life for the better. You are fully capable of change—you've just got to believe it's true!

Embody this Mantra:

1. Breathe in through your nose.

2. Exhale as long as possible until your lungs have completely deflated.

3. Repeat this three times.

4. Before your next breath, say to yourself "My body is constantly helping me"

5. Breathe out until your lungs deflate and recite, "I make better choices for my health"

I Seek Out Healing and It Comes to Me

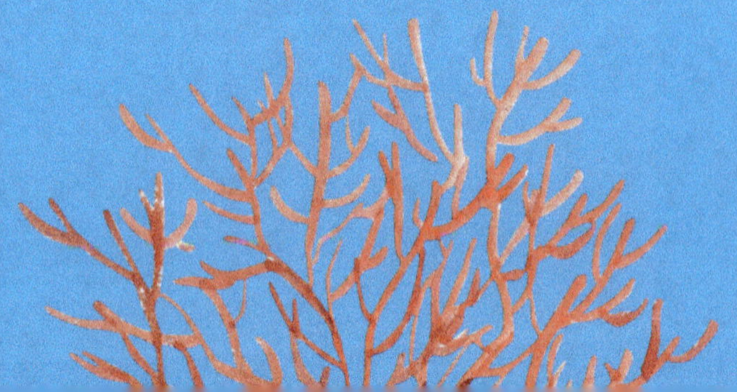

I Seek Out Healing and It Comes to Me

Here's a hack: instead of tucking away your produce in the pantry or closing it away in produce compartments in your fridge (which, is it just me, or are all produce compartments difficult to open anyway?) Why not place most of your fresh produce on your countertop? Get a cool fruit bowl and set it out somewhere in plain sight. This not only adds to the aesthetics of your kitchen, it also serves as a visual cue. The placement of produce in a conspicuous spot primes your brain to choose these foods more often. When you are constantly surrounded by fresh produce, you're more likely to eat them.

Make it easy for yourself to find beneficial foods. And keep in mind, this practice extends beyond produce. You can opt to make your weights more visible, you can keep your yoga mat in an open corner, and you can keep inspirational books on your coffee table. With this mantra, you'll program your subconscious mind to seek out foods and activities that heal and empower you.

Embody this Mantra:

1. Close your eyes.
2. Focus on the air passing in and out of your nostrils, without trying to control the breath.
3. Imagine yourself walking through an orchard until you find a gold apple.
4. Consume the gold apple as you continue breathing with your eyes closed.
5. This represents the foods and activities you seek out to better your life.
6. Imagine your body willing with a gold light for a few more rounds of breath.

My Actions Align with My Words

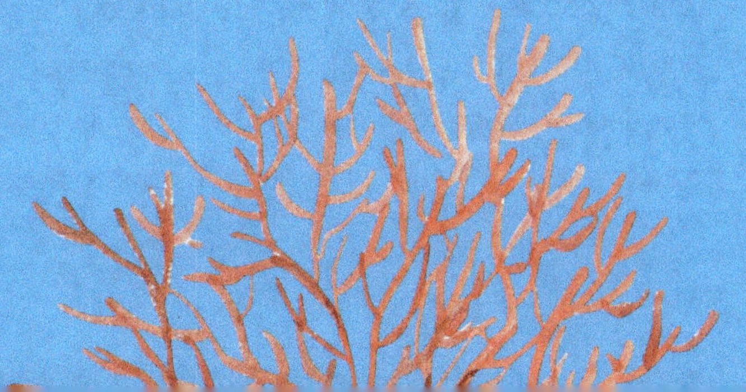

My Actions Align with My Words

While your words have the power to shape your subconscious mind, you've got to take action. If not, your words become meaningless and your subconscious mind will recognize you are lying to it. It's a bit of a Catch-22 situation: On one hand, mantras can spark action; on the other, you may need to first act before you can speak these mantras with confidence and truth.

Let's use the previous mantra as an example: "I seek out healing and it comes to me." When reflecting and reciting this current mantra, My Actions Align with My Words, you could prove that the previous mantra is true—that you do take action and you're more than just talk—by finding evidence that supports this claim. For example, you may remember that time yesterday you reached for grass fed beef instead of packaged ramen noodles (thus proving you seek out healing and that it comes to you). You may remember how you decided to go to the gym instead of laying on the couch watching Netflix. The list goes on. Reflect on the ways your actions have led to the fulfillment of your words.

These mantras have power, but you've got to prove them to be true. Remember: don't be a wet noodle with your words; follow through with passion and vigor.

Embody this Mantra:

1. Take a deep breath.
2. Imagine your ideal self in your mind.
3. Continue breathing and close your eyes.
4. Imagine yourself stepping into, and aligning with, your ideal self.
5. This represents the bridging between your current actions and your words.

You Made It!

Thank you so much for making it through this mantras and affirmations book! I hope it inspires you to make positive changes in your life and fills you with a sense of security in your home: your body. I hope you feel less stressed about the ambiguity and the uncertainty you may be facing. I hope you've adopted a new way of approaching any challenges you may be facing along your healing journey. I hope you become the best version of yourself, all while laughing and loving along the way.

If you found this book useful, please leave a quick review (this is extremely important!) and tell a friend. This way others may also begin to adopt a healing mindset through the use of affirmations and mantras, too.

Other books I've written you might also enjoy:

- Journey On: How to Travel the World - Even If You're Young and Broke

- [Laptop Entrepreneur: Realistic Ways You Can Live the Dream Abroad and Make Money Online](#)

- [The Global Volunteer: Free Travel Opportunities to Help Abroad With Gap Year Programs, The Peace Corps, WWOOF and More](#)

- [Taste Torino: The Local Scoop on Food Paradises, Museums and Secret Sites in Turin](#)

- [Student of the World: How I Earned a Degree Abroad Debt-free and You Can, Too (Study Abroad Guide)](#)

Thanks again for reading. I hope you found, and continue to find, these mantras useful.

About Me

I'm Ryan Scott Shannon, a former fast-paced world traveler turned slow-paced, travel-within type. As of writing this at the end of 2022, I've just finished my master's in work and organizational psychology from the University of Seville (yes, in Spain. Yes, in Spanish). Like just about every other Gen-Zer, I'm trying to escape a corporate career and the 40-hour work week (there's more to life than work and money, right? Where's the time for passions, for rest, for pursuing actualization? For connection?)

While I don't travel as much as I used to, I love teaching people about how to travel cheaply and more authentically via books, ecourses and blog posts. Beyond travel, I'm deeply passionate about psychology after confronting and healing my wounds from my turbulent childhood. I now plan on becoming a licensed professional counselor and plan on writing books that provide people with grounding tools (such as this one).

To see more of my books, click here.

I've also launched Ryan Scott Coffee Table Books which features a collection of children's books, puzzle books and more. Check it out.

Thank You

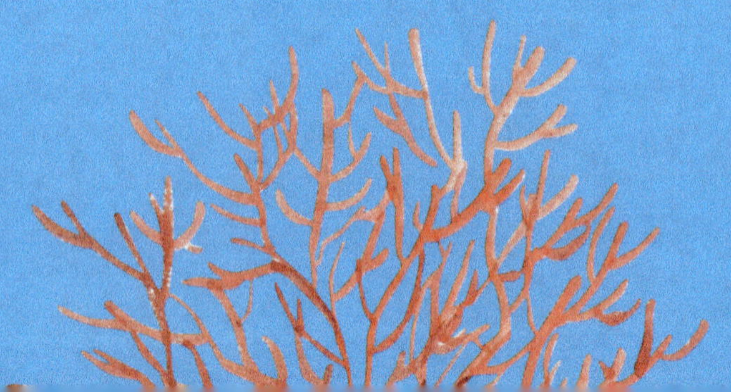

Works Cited

Ai, A. L., et al. "The Role of Private Prayer in Psychological Recovery among Midlife and Aged Patients Following Cardiac Surgery." *The Gerontologist*, vol. 38, no. 5, 1 Oct. 1998, pp. 591–601, 10.1093/geront/38.5.591. Accessed 8 Feb. 2020.

Ando, Yoshinari, et al. "An Era of Single-Cell Genomics Consortia." *Experimental & Molecular Medicine*, vol. 52, no. 9, Sept. 2020, pp. 1409–1418, 10.1038/s12276-020-0409-x. Accessed 2 Mar. 2022.

Barbuzano, Javier. "Understanding How the Intestine Replaces and Repairs Itself." *Harvard*

Gazette, 14 July 2017, news.harvard.edu/gazette/story/2017/07/understanding-how-the-intestine-replaces-and-repairs-itself/.

"Consumer Expenditures in 2020 : BLS Reports: U.S. Bureau of Labor Statistics." *Www.bls.gov,* www.bls.gov/opub/reports/consumer-expenditures/2020/home.htm.

Dempersmier, Jon, and Hei Sook Sul. "Shades of Brown: A Model for Thermogenic Fat." *Frontiers in Endocrinology,* vol. 6, 8 May 2015, 10.3389/fendo.2015.00071. Accessed 6 Dec. 2019.

Fox, Kieran C.R., et al. "Functional Neuroanatomy of Meditation: A Review and Meta-Analysis of 78 Functional Neuroimaging Investigations."

Neuroscience & Biobehavioral Reviews, vol. 65, June 2016, pp. 208–228, 10.1016/j.neubiorev.2016.03.021.

Furness, J. B., et al. "Nutrient Tasting and Signaling Mechanisms in the Gut. II. The Intestine as a Sensory Organ: Neural, Endocrine, and Immune Responses." *The American Journal of Physiology*, vol. 277, no. 5, 1 Nov. 1999, pp. G922-928, pubmed.ncbi.nlm.nih.gov/10564096/, 10.1152/ajpgi.1999.277.5.G922.

Hopper, Susan I., et al. "Effectiveness of Diaphragmatic Breathing for Reducing Physiological and Psychological Stress in Adults." *JBI Database of Systematic Reviews and Implementation Reports*, vol. 17, no. 9,

Sept. 2019, pp. 1855–1876, journals.lww.com/jbisrir/fulltext/2019/09000/effectiveness_of_diaphragmatic_breathing_for.6.aspx, 10.11124/jbisrir-2017-003848.

Hülsheger, Ute R., and Hugo J.E.M. Alberts. "Assessing Facets of Mindfulness in the Context of Work: The Mindfulness@Work Scale as a Work-Specific, Multidimensional Measure of Mindfulness." *Applied Psychology*, 2 Dec. 2020, 10.1111/apps.12297.

Hyland, Patrick K., et al. "Mindfulness at Work: A New Approach to Improving Individual and Organizational Performance." *Industrial and Organizational Psychology*, vol. 8, no. 4, 15 July 2015, pp. 576–602, www.cambridge.org/core/journals/industrial-a

nd-organizational-psychology/article/mindfuln

ess-at-work-a-new-approach-to-improving-ind

ividual-and-organizational-performance/88114

8F1CFDB6C1E2FEECF4962389599,

10.1017/iop.2015.41.

Jacobs, Jeremy M, et al. "Optimism and Longevity beyond Age 85." *The Journals of Gerontology: Series A*, vol. 76, no. 10, 20 Feb. 2021, pp. 1806–1813, 10.1093/gerona/glab051. Accessed 28 Dec. 2022.

Lin, Lifeng. "Bias Caused by Sampling Error in Meta-Analysis with Small Sample Sizes." *PLOS ONE*, vol. 13, no. 9, 13 Sept. 2018, p. e0204056, 10.1371/journal.pone.0204056.

Malaktaris, Anne, et al. "Higher Frequency of Mantram Repetition Practice Is Associated with Enhanced Clinical Benefits among United States Veterans with Posttraumatic Stress Disorder." *European Journal of Psychotraumatology*, vol. 13, no. 1, 10 June 2022, 10.1080/20008198.2022.2078564. Accessed 5 Sept. 2022.

Oman, Doug, et al. "Mantram Repetition as a Portable Mindfulness Practice: Applications during the COVID-19 Pandemic." *Mindfulness*, 16 Nov. 2020, 10.1007/s12671-020-01545-w.

Pascoe, Michaela C., et al. "Psychobiological Mechanisms Underlying the Mood Benefits of Meditation: A Narrative Review." *Comprehensive Psychoneuroendocrinology*, vol. 6, May 2021, p. 100037, 10.1016/j.cpnec.2021.100037. Accessed 24 Mar. 2021.

Schiavon, Cecilia C., et al. "Optimism and Hope in Chronic Disease: A Systematic Review." *Frontiers in Psychology*, vol. 7, 4 Jan. 2017, www.ncbi.nlm.nih.gov/pmc/articles/PMC5209 342/, 10.3389/fpsyg.2016.02022.

"Topic: Pharmaceutical Industry in the U.S." *Www.statista.com*, Statista, 2008, www.statista.com/topics/1719/pharmaceutical -industry/.

Torkamani, Fatemeh, et al. "Effects of Single-Session Group Mantra-Meditation on Salivary Immunoglobulin a and Affective State: A Psychoneuroimmunology Viewpoint."

EXPLORE, vol. 14, no. 2, Mar. 2018, pp. 114–121, 10.1016/j.explore.2017.10.010. Accessed 10 Feb. 2020.

Whitehead, Ross D., et al. "Attractive Skin Coloration: Harnessing Sexual Selection to Improve Diet and Health." *Evolutionary Psychology: An International Journal of Evolutionary Approaches to Psychology and Behavior*, vol. 10, no. 5, 20 Dec. 2012, pp. 842–854, pubmed.ncbi.nlm.nih.gov/23253790/. Accessed 28 Dec. 2022.